Blood Type Diet

Featuring Blood Type Recipes

Valerie Lewis

Table of Contents

Blood Type Diet Introduction

How the Blood Type Affects Diet

The blood type diet has gained in popularity over the past two decades since Dr. Peter D'Adamo first came out with his book *4 Blood Types, 4 Diets, Eat Right 4 Your Type*. While the existence for the need for such a diet remains controversial, you will find strong advocates for it along with their blood type theories. However, at this point and time, there has been no actual scientific or medical research in depth to prove or disprove the theories that a person should stick with a particular diet based solely on their blood type. You can find plenty of support in the theory, just run an internet search about this and see all the websites that stand behind the theory that each blood type needs a certain type of diet.

Since we are discussing the blood type diet, it helps to know the different blood types. We will touch on different types for introduction purposes. First, the blood type is measured from the antigens, the proteins that exist on red blood cells. The blood types O, A, and B are the most common. When a person is blood type A only the type A antigens resides on the surface of the red blood cells. The same goes with type B. Type AB contains both. Blood type O contains neither. There is a third antigen called the Rh factor and it either exists or does not, thus you have the "positive" and "negative" ratings of blood types. Of all the blood types, "O positive" is the most common in the world, with A being a close second.

A naturopathic physician name Peter D' Adamo is the pioneer who first came up with the blood type diet theory, devising an entire diet system around a person's blood type. Many others follow along with the blood type diet theory that the need for a particular diet for each blood type has evolved through the years due to the changes in the environment and in people's methods of obtaining food. He proposes that if a person eats certain foods that go against their blood types they will become weak and the result can show up as diseases and even weight gain.

What the Opposition Says About Blood Type Diets

Those who oppose the blood type diet theory claim they have sufficient evidence supporting their belief; however, again, there is no real scientific or medical research evidence to disprove the theory. Again, do a search for the opposition and find many who support the opposing claim as well. The opposition's main concern is the lack of nutrition balance in the type A and type O diets and the opposition feels that the blood type diets should not be followed for long periods. A newsletter put out by the Harvard Medical School recently cites the lack of scientific evidence for such diets. They question the theory asking what may happen if more than one blood type shows up in a family. This type of reasoning looks at two parents, where one may be (for an example) type O blood, and the other type A. No matter what blood type the child turns out to be, either A or O, it is believed they still have the predisposition of the same behavior as each parent's blood type.

Therefore, it is difficult to assume that a child with a

parent with a different blood type as theirs would benefit from such a strict diet. They further reason that the diet may be beneficial if, and this is a big if, every single family member has the same blood type, and the blood type was handed down through the years from generation to generation. But this is rare, blood types vary as much as skin and hair color.

No diet is one hundred percent great without doing other things to live a healthy lifestyle. Diet is just a piece of the whole puzzle that makes up a complete person. Just choosing sensible foods is a start, meaning to choose fruits and vegetables, lean proteins and to stay away from processed and refined foods. Break bad habits such as smoking and drinking alcohol excessively. Sedentary lifestyles are unhealthy. People need to get up and move around in order to be healthy. Exercise is often overlooked and should be a part of every healthy regimen, even for those with limited physical mobility, being physically active is necessary. If there are physical limitations, seek the help of a physical therapist or a gym instructor to come up with an exercise routine just for you. Dieting, exercising, and healthy lifestyle choices all work together to make a person healthy and whole. Drinking plenty of water with any diet is a must too. Water helps to digest the foods and helps to clean the body. All these things work together, and in doing all of these things together you become healthier faster, reaching your health and fitness goals quicker.

Peter D'Adamo believes that if a person wishes to lose weight they need to eat foods that agree with their blood type, see his book Eat Right for Your Type. D'Adamo would be well served if he would run some actual scientific studies and clinical trials to prove his beliefs. Many people go on his diet and claim it helps, however to draw your own conclusions, you need to test it out for yourself. As with anything having to do with your health, always seek the advice of your healthcare provider before trying any new diet or exercise routine.

Blood Types

As stated above type O is the most common. According to LivingStrong.com 46 % of the population is a type O. 39% is type A and only 11% is type B. Type AB is the rarest and less than 5% of the population has this type.

Type O blood was the original blood type for humanity as believed by Peter D'Adamo. He believes people with type O blood should eat diets rich in proteins and less in glutens. This is how our Stone Age ancestors ate. If you look at the Paleo Diet you will see many similarities to the blood type O diet plan. Type O people of old were hunters and big meat eaters. They did not garden much because they spent all of their time on the hunt. He further states that type A blood came along when people started farming the lands and growing more fruits and vegetables. Type A should focus on grains and vegetarian type foods. Type B is a variation between the two diets. Type AB should avoid legumes and certain grains and seeds. D'Adamo believes that by eating the wrong foods in conjunction with your blood type the result will be excessive body fat.

Peter D'Adamo further believes that blood types affect

the personality. He claims that type O blood people are practical and organized. Type A's are more prone to stress. Type B's are a good cross between the O and A being more adaptable. Type AB is a cross between A and B.

Blood Type O Diet

Peter D'Adamo in his book Eat Right for Your Type claims that following his diet suggestions help to lose weight by eating the right foods and avoiding the wrong foods. The American Academy of Family Physicians recommends for people to use caution with dieting and to make sure to consume well-balanced meals.

This book is specific to the blood type O diet, since type O is the most common. Peter D'Adamo believes that type O blood types are people full of energy. The diet suggested by D'Adamo suggests certain foods that help to build the energy and to reduce weight gain. Please note that all the statements made in this book follow along with the beliefs and suggestions made by Peter D'Adamo. Never take anyone's word about this, do the research for yourself before drawing your own conclusions. Just know that this book does follow with D'Adamo's beliefs and suggestions for the blood type diet plan.

Type Os do well eating a diet high in protein, especially meat. Type Os do not make good vegetarians. They need diets that include plenty of beef, cold-water fish, cod, tuna, rainbow trout, red snapper, halibut, swordfish, and salmon. Eat chicken and shellfish and almonds are okay to eat a couple times a week. A type O person can digest these easily because of the high acidity in their digestive systems.

Type O people often find they gain too much weight when eating foods that contain gluten and other whole grains. Type Os can eat barley and rice with no issues, but should substitute for wheat, corn, and oats.

Nuts such as pecans, pumpkin seeds and walnuts are beneficial to a type O. Some nuts like cashews, peanuts and pistachios and even kidney and navy beans, and lentils should be avoided, as they cause a greater production of stomach acid. Good legumes such as azuki beans, black-eyed peas, and pinto beans are safe to eat. Avoid eggs and egg products too.

Fruits are beneficial especially figs, cherries, prunes, and plums because they help the body to balance the digestive acidity. Citrus fruits like grapefruit, oranges, and tangerines are too high in acid for a type O. Other fruits to avoid are strawberries and blackberries. O blood types benefit from foods that promote thyroid health, because they tend to have more thyroid issues. Avoid these vegetables: Brussels sprouts, cabbage, cauliflower, eggplant and potatoes. Good vegetables are garlic, onions, peppers, pumpkin, okra, turnips, red peppers, leeks, beets, parsnips, Swiss chard, collard greens, and sweet potatoes. Fruits to consume in moderation are apples, grapes, melons, and bananas. Potatoes should be consumed in moderation, as we have found conflicting advice on potatoes for type O blood diet, some say to eat them daily while others say they are not beneficial. Perhaps good advice here would be to try it and see if it affects you in any way.

If you go on the blood type O diet you need to make sure you receive enough calcium and fiber, because the diet is lacking in the foods which naturally contain fiber and calcium. Type O negative needs to eat more chicken, turkey and venison, plus sea vegetables and fish to get the beneficial iodine nutrient. Everything else is the same.

Blood Type A Diet

Type A blood does well on a vegetarian diet enjoying foods such as all vegetables and fruits including legumes and grains. They can eat seafood and soy protein. Foods to avoid are dairy food and red meat. Vegetables they need to avoid are cabbage, eggplant, peppers, potatoes and tomatoes. Type As need to practice exercises that calm and strengthen, much like yoga. This blood type needs to maintain a schedule of food intake, not skipping meals. They do well to eat their protein early in the day and sticking with more vegetables and fruit at night.

Type As do well to eat foods raw and unprocessed. Because they do not do well with animal proteins, they need to eat nuts, legumes, seeds, and tofu. Even though it is recommended to avoid dairy it is okay to consume mozzarella, ricotta, and yogurt in moderation.

Blood Type B Diet

Type B blood, again, does well in the middle of type O and type A, enjoying a little of each foods. They are good to eat both animal protein and dairy. For weight loss, they should focus on eating plenty of eggs, liver, and vegetables. Foods like grains, nuts, and seeds may hinder weight loss, so eat these in moderation. Exercise is more like the type As have to practice, more of a calming but it is okay to do moderate exertion.

Type B's do well eating animal protein and can consume dairy without issues. They should include cottage cheese, cod, halibut, mackerel, milk, flounder, ocean perch, and salmon in their diet.

Vegetables suitable for type B are beets, cabbage, eggplants, bell peppers, broccoli, Brussels sprout, cauliflower, kale, jalapenos, carrots, yams, mustard greens, collard greens, and sweet potatoes.
Fruits suitable for type B are bananas, cranberries, grapes, pineapple, and plums. Type B needs to avoid avocados, coconuts, corn, and tomatoes. Spices to avoid are pepper, ketchup, almond extract, cinnamon, and allspice.

Blood Type AB Diet

Type AB should follow a good cross section of type A and B. AB type can enjoy tofu, seafood, green vegetables, kelp, pineapple, green vegetables, rabbit, lamb, turkey, and mutton. Eggs can be eaten in moderation, a couple time a week, as well as soft dairy cheeses like cottage, mozzarella, and ricotta.

Foods to avoid include corn, polenta, beef, pork, venison, chicken, and buffalo. No pumpkin seeds, poppy seed or sunflower seeds either. No okra, tomatoes, pumpkin, onions, and turnips, either.
Why Wheat Free?

You will notice in these recipes that there is no call for any wheat food. The wheat grown and consumed thousands of years ago is not the same wheat we have today. Because of the interference with mutations and crossings, the wheat plant does not contain the same valuable nutrients it did in years past. Today there is a rise in the number of people suffering from "gluten intolerances and gluten allergies" because of the high protein content found in wheat today. Wheat causes the body to suffer with inflammation from the intolerances.

Even tiny babies are showing wheat intolerances, according to a study by Pharmacia & Upjohn, a Diagnostics CAP System. Other studies show that close to 10 out of every 100 children has a wheat allergy. That is 10% of the population, and it is enough to take notice and do something about it. Avoiding wheat is the best place to start and that is why you will not find wheat ingredients within this recipe book.

Blood Type Recipes

All the recipes in the Blood Type Diet book are inspired from recipes that have been around for a long time. While similar recipes may be found in books and on websites, all the recipes within this book are based on the blood type diet for O, A, B and AB as outlined by Peter D'Adamo in his books on blood type diet and his website as well.

Blood Type O Recipes

Appetizers and Snacks for Blood Type O

Cheese Ball with Herbs

This recipe calls for a tofu cream cheese, but real cream cheese can be used, keeping in mind that dairy products need to be consumed in moderation only.

Makes 1 cheese ball.

Ingredients:

*1 cup of tofu cream cheese (or real cream cheese)
*1 1/2 tablespoon of parsley (dried)
*1 1/2 tablespoon of cilantro (fresh)
*1 tablespoon of chives (fresh snipped)
*2 teaspoons of onions (dried, minced)
*1/2 teaspoon of garlic (minced)
*1/4 teaspoon of thyme (dried)
*1/2 teaspoon of basil (dried)

*1/2 teaspoon of sage (dried)
*couple dashes of hot sauce
*pinch of salt

Directions:

In a bowl mix the 1 cup of tofu cream cheese (or real cream cheese) together with the 1 tablespoon of chives (fresh snipped), 2 teaspoons of onions (dried, minced), 1/2 teaspoon of garlic (minced), 1/4 teaspoon of thyme (dried), 1/2 teaspoon of basil (dried), 1/2 teaspoon of sage (dried), couple dashes of hot sauce, and a pinch of salt. With clean hand, shape into a ball. Mix the dried parsley and cilantro in a bowl then roll the ball in the 1 1/2 tablespoon of parsley (dried) and the 1 1/2 tablespoon of cilantro (fresh) until it is well coated. Cover and refrigerate for at least half an hour before serving. Serve with crackers.

Spinach Dip with Artichokes

This dip is a must have for any party or gathering and goes perfectly with raw vegetables.

Makes a healthy party serving.

Ingredients:

*3 cups of spinach (fresh chopped)
*2 cups of vegetable stock
*1 3/4 cups of artichoke hearts
*1/2 cup of onion (diced)
*1/2 cup of mozzarella (shredded)
*1/3 cup of feta cheese
*1/4 cup of butter (clarified)
*1/4 cup of rice flour
*2 tablespoons of lemon juice
*1 teaspoon of salt
*1/2 teaspoon of garlic (dried)

Directions:

Heat the butter in a saucepan over medium heat. Add the 1/3 cup of diced onion and sauté. Stir in the 1/4 cup of rice flour, creating a nice roux. Pour in the 2 cups of vegetable stock, stirring as you pour. Increase the heat to medium high and stir until it thickens. Sprinkle in the 2 tablespoons of lemon juice, teaspoon of salt, and 1/2 teaspoon of powdered garlic and stir. Add the 3 cups of fresh chopped spinach, 1 3/4 cups of artichoke hearts, 1/2 cup of shredded mozzarella, and the 1/3 cup of feta cheese and stir over low heat until the cheese melts. Serve warm.

Desserts and Treats for Blood Type O

Sugar Cookies

These sugar cookies are gluten free.

Makes 2 dozen.

Ingredients:

*3/4 cup of rice flour (brown)
*1/2 cup of arrowroot flour
*1/2 cup of butter (clarified)
*1/4 cup of honey
*1 egg
*1 tablespoon of almond milk
*1/2 teaspoon of vanilla extract
*1/4 teaspoon of baking powder
*1/8 teaspoon of salt

Directions:

Prep: Preheat the oven to 350 degrees Fahrenheit. In a bowl, add the clarified butter along with the 1/4 cup of honey and the 1/8 teaspoon of salt, whipping it until it is light and fluffy. Stir in the egg, beating it well into the mixture. Add the tablespoon of almond milk and the 1/2 teaspoon of vanilla extract, stirring well. Last, in a separate bowl add the 3/4 cup of rice flour, 1/2 cup of arrowroot flour and the 1/4 teaspoon of baking powder and stir. Gradually stir into the batter. Drop by the teaspoonfuls onto an ungreased cookie sheet, making sure they are at least an inch apart. Bake for about 9 minutes or until golden brown.

Ginger Spice Cookies

This delicious ginger cook is gluten free.

Makes around 3 dozen cookies (depending on the size.)

Ingredients:

*3 cups of almond meal
*2 cups of flour (rice)
*1 cup of agave syrup
*4 eggs
*1 teaspoon of salt
*1 teaspoon of ginger (ground)
*1/2 teaspoon of cloves (ground)

Directions:

Prep: Preheat oven to 300 degrees Fahrenheit. Lightly spray a cookie sheet with cooking spray.

Add the 4 eggs to a bowl and beat. Then stir in the cup of agave syrup. In a separate bowl, add the 3 cups of almond meal, 2 cups of rice flour, teaspoon of salt, teaspoon of ground ginger, and 1/2 teaspoon of ground cloves. Pour the eggs and agave syrup into the dry ingredients and mix well. Drop by the teaspoonful onto the cookie sheet leaving at least 2 inches between each cookie. Bake in hot oven until golden brown, about 10 minutes. Allow to cool for 2 minutes on the cookie sheet before gently removing and placing on a wire rack for complete cooling. Enjoy immediately or store in a cookie jar or an airtight container.

Breads and Rolls for Blood Type O

Rye Bread

This is a lovely rye bread, perfect for eating alone or in a sandwich.

Makes 2 loaves.

Ingredients:

*7 1/2 cups of rye flour
*2 cups of water
*1 egg
*2 tablespoons of molasses
*1 tablespoon of yeast
*1 tablespoon of salt
*1/2 teaspoon of mustard (ground)
*1/4 teaspoon of onion powder

Directions:

Prep: Grease 2 loaf pans with cooking spray.

In a bowl add 7 1/2 cups of rye flour, 2 cups of water, 1

egg, 2 tablespoons of molasses, 1 tablespoon of yeast, 1 tablespoon of salt, 1/2 teaspoon of mustard (ground) and 1/4 teaspoon of onion powder and mix well. The dough will be thick. Spray a sheet of plastic wrap with cooking spray and loosely cover the bowl and place in a warm spot to rise. Allow it to rise to twice its original size and using your fist, punch it down, to release the air. Cover again and let it rise a second time, punching again and then divide the dough into two. Put into the 2 loaf pans and grease hands with butter or cooking spray and pat the dough into the bottom of the pans. Cover again with the sprayed plastic wrap and set in a warm spot for the final rise. Allow the dough to double its size. Before the dough fully reaches its size, preheat the oven to 350 degrees Fahrenheit. Grease a sharp knife and cut a slit down the center of each loaf at the top to make them a split top. Place the loaves in the hot oven and bake for about 40 minutes, until the top is a nice crisp brown.

Dinner Rolls

These dinner rolls makes a great side dish with many entrees, and it is delicious with breakfast or as a quick snack too.

Makes 16 rolls.

Ingredients:

*3 cups of almond flour
*2 cups of flax (ground)
*1 cup of water
*6 eggs
*3 teaspoons of baking powder
*1 teaspoon of baking soda
*3/4 teaspoon of salt

Directions:

Prep: Preheat the oven to 350 degrees Fahrenheit. Spray 16 muffin tins with cooking spray. (Use 2 12-cup muffin pans)
Add the 3 cups of almond flour in a bowl along with the 2 cups of ground flax, 3 teaspoons of baking powder, teaspoon of baking soda and 3/4 teaspoon of salt and

mix. Set aside, in a separate bowl add the 1 cup of water with the 6 eggs, and beat. Gradually pour the egg water into the dry ingredient bowl and mix well. Set aside for 5 minutes, and then evenly spoon the batter into the 16 muffin tins. Bake until the tops turn a golden brown about 20 minutes. Allow to cool before removing from the pan.

Main Dish Recipes for Blood Type O

Meat Loaf

This is a delicious meat loaf made of turkey complete with a sauce topping.

Makes 4 servings.

Ingredients:

*1 1/2 pounds of turkey (ground white meat)
*1 cup of tomato paste
*1 cup of water
*1 cup of onion (sliced thin)
*1 cup of carrots (sliced thin)
*1/2 cup of onions (diced)
*4 seaweed leaves (roasted and ripped into tiny pieces)
*2 eggs (room temperature)
*1/4 teaspoon of garlic (minced)
*salt and pepper to taste

Directions:

Prep: Preheat oven to 400 degrees Fahrenheit. Spray a

small loaf pan with cooking spray. (or use a special meat loaf pan with the drip tray)
Spray a non-stick frying pan with cooking spray and turn heat to medium. Add the cup of sliced thin onions and sliced thin carrots and sauté. Pour into a large bowl, add the 4 ripped seaweed leaves, and toss. Mix in the 1 1/2 pounds of white ground turkey. Beat the eggs in a cup and add to the meat mixure, with hands knead until mixed. Sprinkle salt and pepper. Add to the loaf pan. In a small bowl, mix the cup of tomato paste, cup of water, 1/2 cup of dice onions, and the 1/4 teaspoon of minced garlic. Poke holes in the top of the meatloaf with your finger and then pour the tomato sauce over the top, filling the holes and covering the top. Meat loaf is done when a meat thermometer inserted in the middle reads 165 degrees Fahrenheit. Start checking in 15 minutes, then check every 5 minutes. Allow to cool, turn out onto a platter and slice and serve.

Chicken and Bean Stew

When the palate is craving a delicious comfort food, reach for this recipe and warm up to a hot steaming bowl of stew. This goes well with the Dinner Rolls.

Makes 4 servings.

Ingredients:

*2 cups of chicken broth
*1 1/2 cups of chicken breasts (cut into small chunks)
*1 1/2 cups of carrots (chopped)
*1 cup of water
*1 cup of beans (adzuki)
*1 cup of celery (chopped)
*3/4 cup of onions (sliced and cut)
*3 tablespoons of olive oil (divided)
*1 1/2 teaspoons of garlic (minced)
*1 bay leaf
*salt and pepper to taste

Directions:

Prep: Sort and wash the cup of adzuki beans and put in a bowl. Add enough water to cover the beans, about 1/2 inches above. Soak overnight.

Pour the water from the beans, add beans to a pot, and cover again with water. Place on stove on high temperature and bring to a boil. Turn down to low and cook for an hour, watching the water, making sure the beans stay covered in water. If you add more water, add hot water. Meanwhile, add the 2 tablespoons of olive oil to a skillet and turn heat to medium. Add the chunked chicken and cook until just done, careful not to "fry" it. Carefully remove the chicken from the skillet, placing it in a bowl, set aside. Keep the heat on the skillet at medium and add the final tablespoon of olive oil. Add the 3/4 cup of sliced cut onion and the 1 1/2 teaspoons of minced garlic and sauté. Place the 1 1/2 cups of chopped carrots and the cup of chopped celery in a small saucepan and cover with water. Place on high heat, bring to a boil, and boil for 5 minutes. Remove from heat and drain the water. In a large pan add the adzuki beans, browned chicken, sautéed onions and garlic, cooked carrots and celery, 2 cups of chicken broth, 1 cup of water, the bay leaf and salt and pepper. Bring to a quick boil on high heat, turn to low, and cook for about half an hour. Remove the bay leaf and allow cooling slightly before serving.

Beef and Gravy

This makes a great dish to serve over steamed vegetables or rice.

Makes 6 servings.

Ingredients:

*2 pounds of beef (use whatever cut you like, slice into bite-sized cubes)
*1 3/4 cups of beef broth
*1/3 cup of rice flour
*1/4 cup of olive oil
*1/4 cup of onion (diced)
*2 tablespoons of Worcestershire sauce
*1 tablespoon of tamari
*1/2 teaspoon of pepper
*1/2 teaspoon of salt
*1/2 teaspoon of garlic (minced)

Directions:

Put the bite-sized beef in a large zipper bag along with the 1/3 cup of rice flour. Close the bag and shake to coat each piece of beef. Pour the 1/4 cup of olive oil in a skillet and heat to medium high, place the flour coated beef in the hot oil and brown the beef. Do this in batches so all pieces will be well done. Place on a platter and add the 1/4 cup of diced onion to the hot oil and the 1/2 teaspoon of mince garlic and sauté. If the oil is dried, pour in a little of the beef broth. Pour in the remainder of the beef broth once the onions are done along with the 2 tablespoons of Worcestershire sauce, tablespoon of tamari, 1/2 teaspoons of the pepper and salt. Turn the heat to low, cover and simmer for about 2 hours, or until the "gravy" is thick and bubbly. Pour the gravy over the beef, or add the beef and spoon it together to serve.

Side Dish Recipes for Blood Type O

Green Rice Stir Fry

This is an excellent side dish to go well with a meaty protein rich main dish.

Makes 2 large or 4 small servings.

Ingredients:

*1 cup of kale (chopped)
*3/4 cup of onion (red - chopped)
*3/4 cup of rice (basmati)
*1/2 cup of seaweed
*2 tablespoons of olive oil
*1 tablespoon of agave syrup
*1/2 tablespoon of turmeric
*1/4 tablespoon of coriander
*1/4 tablespoon of cayenne
*5 teaspoons of garlic (minced)

Directions:

Prep: Cook the 3/4 cup of basmati rice according to

package directions.

Add the 2 tablespoons of olive oil to a frying pan and heat to medium. Stir in the 3/4 cup of chopped red onion, 1/2 cup of seaweed, and the 5 teaspoons of minced garlic and sauté. Add the 3/4 cup of cooked basmati rice with the tablespoon of agave syrup, 1/2 tablespoon of turmeric, 1/4 tablespoon of coriander and the 1/4 tablespoon of cayenne and continue cooking for another 10 minutes. Toss in the cup of chopped kale at the last minute, and stir until wilted. Serve immediately with a meat main dish.

Potato Salad

Potato salad goes with many meat dishes.

Makes 4 servings.

Ingredients:

*8 cups of potatoes (cubed)
*2 cups of celery (sliced)
*2 cups of mayonnaise
*1 cup of onion (minced
*4 eggs
*4 tablespoons of vinegar
*3 teaspoons of salt
*2 teaspoons of sugar
*1/2 teaspoon of pepper

Directions:

Prep: Boil the 4 eggs to "hard boiled." Cook the 8 cups of potatoes until tender enough to eat, but not mashed.

In a small bowl, mix the 2 cups of mayonnaise, 4 tablespoons of vinegar, 3 teaspoons of salt, 2 teaspoons of sugar, and 1/2 teaspoon of pepper. In a large bowl, add the 4 minced hard-boiled eggs along with the 8 cups of cooked cubed potatoes, 2 cups of sliced celery, and the cup of minced onion. Toss, then pour the mayonnaise mixture and gently stir to coat well. Serve with meal.

Blood Type A Recipes

Appetizers and Snacks

Sardine Salad Spread

This delicious spread is great on crackers or bread.

Makes 2 sandwiches or spread for 8 crackers.

Ingredients:

*2 cans of sardines (water packed 8 oz.)
*juice from one lemon
*1 cup of onions (diced)
*1 cup of bell pepper (diced)
*4 tablespoons of tahini
*2 tablespoons of olive oil
*4 teaspoons of garlic (minced)
*2 teaspoons of cumin
*1 teaspoon of salt

Directions:

Open the 2 cans of sardines and drain the water. Add to a bowl and mash. Mix in the 4 tablespoons of tahini, 4 teaspoons of minced garlic, 2 teaspoons of cumin and the teaspoon of salt. Heat the 2 tablespoons of olive oil in a skillet over medium heat. Add the cup of diced onions and the cup of diced bell pepper and sauté. Mix the vegetables in with the mashed sardines. Stir in the juice of the lemon. Refrigerate until chilled then spread on bread or crackers.

Fried Asparagus

Fried asparagus makes great appetizers and may be used in place of French fries as well.

Makes 4 servings.

Ingredients:

*16 sprigs of asparagus
*olive oil
*salt

Directions:

Prep: Line a baking sheet with foil. Preheat the oven to broil.

Cut the asparagus for cooking by snipping the ends. Lay the asparagus on the lined baking sheet, drizzle with olive oil then sprinkle with salt. Place under the broiler for 8 minutes. Turn the asparagus sprigs over and bake for another 4 minutes. Enjoy.

Desserts and Treats for Blood Type A

Blue-Cranberry Muffins

A delicious muffin that is good as a dessert or even for breakfast or brunch.

Makes 2 dozen muffins.

Ingredients:

*3 cups of flour (spelt)
*1 1/2 cups of blueberries (frozen)
*1 1/2 cups of cranberries (chopped)
*1 cup of olive oil
*1 cup of honey
*4 eggs
*4 teaspoons of lime juice
*1 1/2 teaspoons of baking soda
*1 teaspoon of vanilla

Directions:

Prep: Preheat oven to 350 degrees Fahrenheit. Line 24 muffin tins with cupcake liners.

Add the 3 cups of spelt flour to a bowl along with the 1 1/2 teaspoons of baking soda and mix. Set aside. In a separate bowl, add the 4 eggs and beat, then add the cup of olive oil, cup of honey, 4 teaspoons of lime juice and the teaspoon of vanilla. Mix well, and gradually add in the dry ingredients. Equally spoon the batter into the 24 lined muffin tins. Bake until tops turn a golden brown, about 25 minutes.

Fudge Cookies

This delicious recipe for cookies calls for carob instead of cocoa and non-wheat flours.

Makes 3 dozen cookies.

Ingredients:

*1 3/4 cups of flour (spelt)
*1/2 cup of carob powder
*1/2 cup of walnuts (chopped)
*1/2 cup of honey
*1/2 cup of soy milk
*1/3 cup of olive oil
*1 1/2 teaspoons of baking powder
*1/4 teaspoon of salt

Directions:

Prep: Preheat the oven to 350 degrees Fahrenheit.

Mix the 1 3/4 cups of spelt flour with the 1/2 cup of carob powder, 1 1/2 teaspoons of baking powder, and the 1/4 teaspoon of salt. In a separate bowl, add the1/2 cup of honey, 1/2 cup of soy milk, 1/3 cup of olive oil and stir. Gradually add the dry ingredients, and then gently fold in the 1/2 cup of chopped walnuts. Drop by the teaspoonful onto an ungreased baking sheet. Bake for 8 minutes. Allow to cool for 2 minutes on the cookie sheet before transferring to a wire rack for complete cooling.

Breads and Rolls for Blood Type A

Rice Bread

This is a delicate light bread that goes well with meals.

Makes one round loaf.

Ingredients:

*1 cup of flour (rice)
*1 cup of soy milk
*2 eggs
*2 teaspoons of baking powder
*1 teaspoon of basil (dried)
*1 teaspoon of oregano (dried)
*1/4 teaspoon of salt

Directions:

Prep: Add the cup of rice flour in a bowl along with the cup of soy milk and sit for an hour. Next in a separate bowl, add just the egg whites reserving the yolks. With a whisk beat the egg whites until peaks form. Add the rice flour and milk mixture to the egg whites and gently stir.

Mix in the 2 egg yolks along with the 2 teaspoons of baking powder, teaspoon of dried basil, teaspoon of dried oregano and the 1/4 teaspoon of salt. Next, spray the top of a double boiler with cooking spray and place the dough in the top of it. Cover the top with foil, making a tent to allow the bread to rise as it cooks. Set the stove to produce a gentle boil in the pan of water beneath the bread. Make sure the foil covers the bread not to allow water to get into the top pan. Allow the water to boil gently for 80 minutes under the bread pan. Remove the pan from the double boiler and let it cool on a wire rack for about 10 minutes. Turn out onto a platter and allow cooling completely. Serve immediately, or store in an airtight container for a couple of days.

Buttermilk Biscuits

Biscuits go well with any meal from breakfast through supper.
Makes a dozen biscuits.

Ingredients:

*2 cups of flour (spelt)
*1 cup of buttermilk
*1 tablespoon of baking powder
*1/4 teaspoon of salt

Directions:

Prep: Preheat oven to 425 degrees Fahrenheit. Lightly spray a baking sheet with cooking spray.

Add the 2 cup of spelt flour along with the tablespoon of baking powder and 1/4 teaspoon of salt to a bowl and mix. Stir in the cup of buttermilk. Evenly drop by spoonfuls onto the baking sheet making a dozen biscuits. Bake until golden brown, around 13 minutes.

Main Dish Recipes Side Dish Recipes for Blood Type A

Italian Chicken Breasts

This chicken dish makes an Italian treat that all will love.

Makes 6 servings.

Ingredients:

*6 chicken breast halves (boneless and skinless)
*1 cup of bread crumbs (fine)
*1/4 cup of Romano cheese (grated)
*3 tablespoons of oregano (dried)
*2 tablespoons of kelp (powder)

Directions:

Prep: Preheat oven to 375 degrees Fahrenheit. In a shallow dish, mix the cup of fine breadcrumbs with the 1/4 cup of grated Romano cheese, 3 tablespoons of dried oregano, and the 2 tablespoons of kelp powder. Rinse the chicken breast halves, and then roll through the breadcrumb mixture. Arrange the breasts in a baking dish, not overlapping. Bake for about an hour, checking to make sure the temperature reaches 165 degrees Fahrenheit with a meat thermometer inserted into the middle.

Salmon with Eggplant

Salmon is so beneficial, chocked full of nutrients. Try this delicious dish, which features eggplant.

Makes 4 servings.

Ingredients:

*1 pound of salmon (fillet - skinless)
*1/2 cup of basil leaves (fresh)
*1/2 cup of olive oil (extra virgin)
*10 parsley sprigs (fresh)
*3 tablespoons of pine nuts
*1 tablespoon of garlic (minced) +1 teaspoon
*1 teaspoon of olive oil
*salt to taste

Directions:

Prep: Preheat the oven to 350 degrees Fahrenheit.

Cut the salmon fillets into 4 servings. Rinse with water and dry with a paper towel. Place the salmon fillets in a glass baking dish and sprinkle the teaspoon of olive oil along with the tablespoon of minced garlic. Make the pesto by adding these ingredients into a food processor or blender: 3 tablespoons of pine nuts and 1 teaspoon of minced garlic. Chop the two ingredients. Add the 1/2 cup of fresh basil leaves, 10 fresh parsley sprigs and the 1/2 cup of extra virgin olive oil and continue to "chop" until it forms pesto. Sprinkle with salt to taste. Spread the pesto over the top of the salmon. Bake in the oven for 15 minutes, uncovered. Serve immediately.

Green Pasta Dish

This is a perfect dish for vegetarians as well as all blood types, especially type A.

Makes 4 servings.

Ingredients:

*1 pound of artichoke pasta
*1 pound of raw spinach (washed and chopped)
*1 bunch of Swiss chard (washed and chopped and trimmed)
*1 cup of leeks (sliced)
*1/4 cup of olive oil
*1 teaspoon of garlic (minced)
*salt to taste
*Romano cheese to taste

Directions:

Pour water in a large pot and bring to a boil on the stove. Add the artichoke pasta and cook according to package directions. In a large frying pan add the 1/4 cup of olive oil and cook the cup of sliced leeks until they tenderize. Add the teaspoon of minced garlic and cook for another minute. Toss in the pound of raw spinach and the bunch of Swiss chard and cook until the greens wilt and are fully cooked through. Toss in some salt and Romano cheese and serve.

Side Dish Recipes for Blood Type A

Spicy Beets and Vegetables

This side dish gives beneficial nutrients from the beets, carrots, and turnips.

Makes 4 servings.

Ingredients:

*6 beets (greens included, peeled and cubed)
*2 turnips (fresh. peeled and cubed)
*4 cups of carrots (chopped)
*1/2 cup of onion (yellow chopped)
*2 tablespoons of tamari
*1/2 teaspoon of allspice
*1/2 teaspoon of cinnamon (ground)
*1/4 teaspoon of ginger (ground)
*1/4 teaspoon of cloves
*olive oil
*salt to taste

Directions:

Add the 6 chopped and peeled beets along with the 4 cups of chopped carrots to a pot of boiling water. Salt the water. Boil for 10 minutes to soften. Drain the water and set to the side. Add a little olive oil to a skillet and turn to medium heat, add the 1/2 cup of chopped yellow onion and sauté. Add the 2 peeled and cubed turnips along with the 2 tablespoons of tamari, 1/2 teaspoon of allspice, 1/2 teaspoon of ground cinnamon, 1/4 teaspoon of ground ginger, and the 1/4 teaspoon of cloves. Sauté for another 5 minutes. Pour in the beet and carrot mixture and continue cooking for another 7 minutes. Salt to taste.

Rice Stuffing

This is an excellent side dish to turkey or chicken.

Makes about 4 servings.

Ingredients:

*2 cup of rice (cooked)
*1/2 cup of celery (chopped, celery leaves included)
*1/4 cup of onion (chopped)
*1 tablespoon of parsley (dried)
*1 tablespoon of poultry seasoning (add more if desired)
*salt to taste
*olive oil

Directions:

Pour enough olive oil to coat the bottom of a skillet and heat to medium. Add the 1/2 cup of chopped celery and celery leaves with the 1/4 cup of chopped onion). Sprinkle in the tablespoon of dried parsley and the poultry seasoning. Stir in the rice and add extra olive oil if needed to keep it moist. Salt to taste. Stir until heated through.

Blood Type B Recipes

Appetizers and Snacks for Blood Type B

Potato Chips

These are not your average potato chips, they are made from sweet potatoes.

Makes 4 servings.

Ingredients:

*4 sweet potatoes (sliced very thin)
*salt to taste
*cayenne pepper to taste

Directions:

Prep: Preheat oven to 450 degrees. Spray a cookie sheet with cooking spray. (may need 2 cookie sheets)
Spread the sweet potato slices on a single layer on the

sprayed cookie sheet. Bake until the slices turn golden and crisp. It only takes a couple of minutes. Sprinkle salt and cayenne pepper while hot, serve immediately. Store in an airtight container. May spread and reheat for 2 minutes after storage.

Meatballs a la Turkey

Meatballs make a great appetizer, just skewer with a toothpick, place on a platter and you have a hit.

Makes 2 pounds of meatballs.

Ingredients:

*2 pounds of turkey (ground)
*1 cup of bread crumbs
*1 cup of cranberries (dried and chopped)
*1/2 cup of onion (minced)
*1/2 cup of parsley (fresh chopped)
*1 1/2 teaspoon of garlic (minced)
*salt to taste
*pepper to taste

Directions:

Prep: Preheat oven to 400 degrees Fahrenheit. Spray a broiler pan with cooking spray.

In a large bowl add the 2 pounds of turkey, then add the 1 cup of bread crumbs, 1 cup of cranberries, dried and chopped), 1/2 cup of onion (minced), 1/2 cup of parsley (fresh chopped), 1 1/2 teaspoon of garlic (minced), salt to taste, and the pepper to taste. With hands, mix all the ingredients well. Shape into 1-inch meatballs. Place on the greased broiler pan and back until the tops brown, turn the meatballs and brown on all sides. Serve with toothpicks and dip into favorite dipping sauce, or with pasta and sauce.

Desserts and Treats for Blood Type B

Chocolate Chip Cookies

Most people enjoy a good chocolate chip cookie, these are very good.

Makes 2 dozen cookies.

Ingredients:

*2 cups of rice flour (brown)
*1 cup of honey
*1 cup of canola oil
*1/2 cup of potato flour
*1/2 cup of water
*1/2 cup of chocolate chips
*2 eggs
*4 teaspoons of baking powder
*2 teaspoons of vanilla extract
*1 teaspoon of baking soda
*2 dashes of stevia

Directions:

Prep: Preheat oven to 375 degrees Fahrenheit.

Add the 2 eggs to a large bowl and beat and then add in the 1 cup of honey, 1 cup of canola oil, 2 teaspoons of vanilla extract, and the 2 dashes of stevia and stir well. In a separate bowl, mix the 2 cups of brown rice flour, 1/2 cup of potato flour, 4 teaspoons of baking powder, and the teaspoon of baking soda. Gradually add the dry ingredients into the batter. Fold in the 1/2 cup of chocolate chips. Using greased hands make 2 dozen balls and place on a cookie sheet 2 inches apart. Bake in oven for about 11 minutes, until light golden brown. Allow to cool on pan for 2 minutes, then remove to wire rack until completely cooled.

CranNut Cake

This is a delicious small cake, perfect to satisify the sweet tooth.
Makes one 13x9 or two98 inch round cakes.

Ingredients:

*2 cups of rice flour
*2 cups of flax meal
*2 cups of hot water
*2 cups of cranberries
*2 cups of walnuts
*1 1/4 cup of honey
*2 tablespoons of ghee
*2 tablespoons of black strap molasses
*2 teaspoons of baking soda
*1 teaspoon of cloves

Directions:

Prep: Preheat oven to 350 degrees Fahrenheit. Spray the baking pan(s) with cooking spray.

In a bowl mix the 2 cups of rice flour, 2 cups of flax meal with the 2 cups of hot water. Stir and set aside for 10 minutes. In a separate bowl add the 1 1/4 cup of honey, 2 tablespoons of ghee, 2 tablespoons of black strap molasses, 2 teaspoons of baking soda, and the teaspoon of cloves and stir. Mix in the flours and water bowl. Fold in the 2 cups each of the cranberries and the walnuts. If you desire, chop the cranberries and nuts first. Pour the thick batter into the prepared pan(s) and bake for around 25 minutes, until the top turns a nice golden brown. You may frost with your favorite frosting.

Breads and Rolls for Blood Type B

Loaf of Bread

This is a great bread to slice and eat with sandwiches or to make toast.

Makes one loaf of bread.

Ingredients:

*1 cup of hot water
*1 cup of cannellini bean flour
*1 cup of rice flour (brown)
*3/4 cup of almond milk
*1/2 cup of flax meal
*1/2 cup of arrowroot
*3 eggs
*3 tablespoons of olive oil
*1 tablespoon of vinegar (apple cider)
*1 tablespoon of honey + 1 teaspoon
*1 tablespoon of yeast
*2 teaspoons of lecithin
*1 1/2 teaspoon of salt

Directions:

Prep: Heat the oven to 200 degrees Fahrenheit, then turn the oven off and leave the oven door open just a touch to allow the heat to escape.

Add the teaspoon of honey and the tablespoon of honey to the cup of hot water, stir, and set aside. Add the cups of cannellini bean flour, brown rice flour, 1/2 cup of flax meal, 1/2 cup of arrowroot, 2 teaspoons of lecithin, and 1 1/2 teaspoons of salt to a bowl and stir. In a separate bowl beat the 3 eggs and add the 3/4 cup of almond milk, 3 tablespoons of olive oil, tablespoon of apple cider vinegar, and the tablespoon of honey and stir well. Gradually add the dry ingredients into the wet ingredients, including the yeast and honey water. Beat with an electric beater for one minute. Prepare the loaf pan by spraying with cooking spray and place a sheet of parchment paper in the bottom. Place the dough in the prepared loaf pan. Place a towel over the loaf pan and place the pan in the oven to let it rise for about an hour. The loaf is ready when it rises just over the top of the loaf pan. Remove the cloth and turn the oven to 350 degrees Fahrenheit. Bake until the top turns a nice golden brown, about 45 minutes.

Dinner Rolls for Type B

These rolls make a delicious bread side dish for many meals.

Makes 15 rolls.

Ingredients:

*6 cups of spelt flour (white)
*2 cups of warm water (just shy of 2 cups, a smidgen less)
*1/3 cup of cold water
*3 teaspoons of yeast
*1 1/2 tablespoons of honey
*1 1/2 tablespoons of olive oil
*1 3/4 teaspoons of salt
*1 1/2 teaspoon of arrowroot

Directions:

Add the 6 cups of white spelt flour with the 3 teaspoons of yeast, and the 1 3/4 teaspoons of salt, and stir in the "just shy of" 2 cups of warm water, 1 1/2 tablespoons of honey, and the 1 1/2 tablespoons of olive oil. Line a baking sheet (or two) with parchment paper. With greased hands make 15 oval shaped "rolls" and place on the parchment paper with about 2 inches between each roll. Spray a piece of plastic wrap with cooking spray and loosely cover the rolls. Set aside to rise to desired size, about an hour. Preheat oven to 350 degrees Fahrenheit. Remove the plastic wrap (carefully). Mix the 1 1/2 teaspoons of arrowroot into the 1/3 cup of cold water. Brush the tops of the rolls with the mixture. Place the rolls in the hot oven and bake until golden brown, around half an hour.

Main Dish Recipes for Blood Type B

Fried Chicken Steak

This is a delicious main entree.

Makes 4 servings.

Ingredients:

*1 pound of beef cube steak
*1/2 cup of spelt flour
*1/4 cup of soy milk
*1 egg
*2 tablespoons of olive oil (extra virgin)
*garlic salt to taste
*crushed red peppers to taste

Directions:

Add the 2 tablespoons of olive oil to a skillet and heat to medium high. In a shallow bowl add the egg and beat, then add the soy milk and mix well with a whisk. In a separate shallow bowl add the 1/2 cup of spelt flour and sprinkle with the garlic salt and crushed red peppers. Cut the beef cube steak into four equal portions. Dip each piece of beef cube steak into the egg mixture, then drag through the flour mixture and place in the skillet and cook for at least 3 minutes. Turn over and cook an additional three minutes.

Steak and Mushrooms

Here is another great recipe using your favorite cut of lean steak.

Makes 2 large servings or 4 small servings.

Ingredients:

*1 to 2 pounds of steak (your favorite cut, lean)
*2 cups of greens (mustard, turnip, broccoli, etc. your choice)
*1 cup of carrots (chopped)
*1 cup of vegetable broth
*1 cup of Portobello mushrooms (chopped)
*1/4 cup of parsley (fresh minced)
*2 tablespoons of lime juice
*2 tablespoons of olive oil
*1 tablespoon of pine nuts
*1 tablespoon of rice flour
*1 tablespoon of garlic (minced)
*1 tablespoon of honey
*1 teaspoon of mustard (prepared)
*salt to taste
*pepper to taste

Directions:

Put the 2 cups of greens and the chopped cup of carrots into a steamer and let them steam while preparing the rest. Cook the steak in your favorite method (grill, broiler, frying pan) and salt and pepper. Add the 2 tablespoons of olive oil to a skillet and heat to medium. Add the tablespoon of minced garlic and the cup of chopped Portobello mushrooms and sauté. Stir in the tablespoon of rice flour to make a rue. Pour in the cup of vegetable broth, stirring as you pour. Add the 2 tablespoons of lime juice, tablespoon of honey and teaspoon of prepared mustard, stirring while the gravy thickens. Add salt and pepper if desired. Put the dish together by spooning a serving of vegetables on the plate; place the cooked meat on top of the steamed vegetables. Pour the gravy over the meat. Garnish with a sprinkling of fresh minced parsley and a few pine nuts. Add more salt and pepper and enjoy.

Baked Italian Meatballs

This is a delicious main course that goes well with pasta and vegetables.

Makes 6 servings.

Ingredients:

*2 pounds of ground beef (lean)
*1 cup of bread crumbs (fine)
*1/2 cup of Romano cheese (pecorino)
*1/2 cup of parsley (fresh chopped)
*1/4 cup of soy milk
*2 eggs
*1 tablespoon of basil leaf (dried)
*3 teaspoons of garlic (minced)
*salt to taste
*pepper to taste

Directions:

Prep: Preheat the oven to 350 degrees Fahrenheit.

Beat the 2 eggs then add to a large bowl along with the remaining ingredients. With hands, combine the 2 pounds of ground beef (lean),1 cup of bread crumbs (fine), 1/2 cup of Romano cheese (pecorino), 1/2 cup of parsley (fresh chopped), 1/4 cup of soy milk, 1 tablespoon of basil leaf (dried), and the 3 teaspoons of garlic (minced). Salt and pepper the mixture and combine well. Roll the meat mixture into whatever size meatballs you want. The larger they are the longer it takes to cook. Line a baking sheet with foil and place the meatballs in a single layer. Bake in the oven for 20 to 30 minutes, turning the meatballs every 5 to 10 minutes to brown on all sides.

Side Dish Recipes for Blood Type B

Roasted Sweet Potatoes

Sweet potatoes go well with so many different main entrees. They also make a great sweet snack.

Makes 4 servings.

Ingredients:

*2 sweet potatoes (cut in half lengthwise)
*1/4 cup of olive oil
*salt to taste

Directions:

Prep: Preheat the oven to 400 degrees Fahrenheit. Cover a baking sheet with foil.

Brush the oil over the tops of the sweet potato halves and sprinkle with salt. Bake for half an hour, the peel will be crisp and the top a golden brown.

Green Beets

Do not let the name full you, the green means the tops of the beets, but the meat of the beets are still a deep red. This is a wonderful side dish that goes well with so many foods, it also acts as a soup.

Makes 4 servings.

Ingredients:

*4 cups of beets and greens (washed and chopped greens, thin sliced beets)
*2 cups of vegetable broth
*4 tablespoons of olive oil

Directions:

In a stockpot, pout the 4 tablespoons of olive oil and heat to medium high. Stir in the beets until heated, stir in the greens, and then add the 2 cups of vegetable broth. Cover and continue to simmer until the beets are tender enough to eat.

Blood Type AB Recipes

Appetizers and Snacks for Blood Type AB

Tortilla Cracker Chips

Everyone deserves a chippy or cracker snack, to eat with your favorite spread or dip. These can be both.

Makes 4 servings. (more or less depending on how many you want to eat in one sitting, because these are so good you cannot have just one!)

Ingredients:

*2 cups of amaranth flour
*6 tablespoons of water (or more)
*2 tablespoons of olive oil
*salt to taste

Directions:

Prep: Preheat oven to 350 degrees Fahrenheit.

Pour the 2 cups of amaranth flour into a bowl and add the 6 tablespoons of water to form a nice dough. Add more water if needed. With hands (grease with olive oil if needed or pat with amaranth flour) form into a dough ball. Divide into eight portions. Place the dough balls onto a floured surface and roll into flat "tortillas". Keep the rolling pin floured as well as the surface. Place 4 tortillas onto two baking sheets. Brush the olive oil on the tops of the tortillas. Sprinkle with salt. Bake until the tortillas are a golden brown and crisp like a cracker or chip, about 7 minutes.

Veggies and Goat's Cheese Dip

This is a great dip for that tortilla cracker chips recipe or for any sliced or diced raw vegetable.

Makes a little over a cup (enough to put in a bowl and enjoy at a small dinner party or to eat alone!)

Ingredients:

*1 cup of goat's cheese
*2 tablespoons of lemon juice
*2 tablespoons of parsley (dried)
*1 tablespoon of sour cream
*1 teaspoon of ginger (ground)
*1 teaspoon of coriander (ground)
*1/2 teaspoon of garlic (minced)
*dash of paprika

Directions:

Prep: Allow the goat's cheese to warm up to room temperature.

Add the cup of goat's cheese to a bowl, pour the 2 tablespoons of lemon juice in, and mash the cheese and juice together. Add the 2 tablespoons o dried parsley, tablespoon of sour cream, teaspoon of ground ginger, teaspoon of ground coriander, and the 1/2 teaspoon of minced garlic and mix well. Sprinkle paprika over the top and serve with raw vegetables, crackers, or chips.

Desserts and Treats for Blood Type AB

Coffee Cake

This cake makes a wonderful dessert but can make a great breakfast and snack too.

Makes one 8x8 square or 8 inch round cake.

Ingredients:

*1 cup of millet flour
*1 1/4 cup of rice flour (brown) (divided)
*3/4 cup of water + more as needed
*1/3 cup of rice flour (sweet)
*1/4 cup of water (boiling hot)
*1/4 cup of almonds (ground)
*1 packet of yeast
*3 tablespoons of olive oil
*4 tablespoons of agave syrup (divided)
*1 tablespoon of flax meal (golden)
*1 tablespoon f lemon juice
*2 teaspoons of canola oil
*1/2 teaspoon of baking soda
*3/4 teaspoon of salt (divided)

Directions:

Prep: Preheat oven to 350 degrees Fahrenheit. Lightly spray an 8x8 or 8-inch round pan with cooking spray.

In a bowl, combine 1 cup of millet flour, 1 cup of brown rice flour, 1/3 cup of sweet rice flour, and the packet of yeast. In a separate bowl, combine the 3/4 cup of water, 3 tablespoons of olive oil, 2 tablespoons of agave syrup, and the tablespoon of lemon juice. Add the tablespoon of golden flax meal to the 1/4 cup of boiling water. Pour the water, flax meal into the wet ingredients and stir. Gently add the dry ingredients into the batter and stir. Pour the batter into the prepared pan. In a small bowl, combine the 1/4 cup of ground almonds, 1/4 cup of rice flour, 2 tablespoons of agave syrup, and the 2 teaspoons of canola oil. Sprinkle over the top of the batter in the pan do not stir. Bake until the top turns a golden brown, about 20 minutes.

Nutty Baked Yellow Delicious Apples

For apple lovers this is a delicious apple desert.

Makes 4 servings.

Ingredients:

*4 yellow delicious apples (large)
*1 cup of apple juice
*1 cup of yogurt (plain)
*1/2 cup of almond butter (creamy)
*1/3 cup of raisins
*1 tablespoon of honey
*1 1/2 teaspoons of vanilla extract
*1/2 teaspoon of cinnamon (ground)
*1/4 teaspoon of nutmeg (ground)

Directions:

Prep: Preheat oven to 375 degrees Fahrenheit.

In a bowl, combine the 1/2 cup of creamy almond butter, 1/3 cup of raisins, 1 1/2 teaspoons of vanilla extract, 1/2 teaspoon of ground cinnamon, 3/4 tablespoon of apple juice with the 1/4 teaspoon of ground nutmeg. Carefully cut the core from the top of the apple, leaving the bottom intact, creating a narrow bowl inside the apple. Fill each apple with the almond butter mixture. Place the 4 apples in a baking dish. Pour the remainder from the cup of apple juice into the dish. Carefully place in the oven and bake for 20 minutes. While baking, mix the cup of plain yogurt with the tablespoon of honey. To serve place a baked apple on a plate or shallow bowl and drizzle the yogurt sauce over the top.

Breads and Rolls for Blood Type AB

Zucchini Bread

This is your classic zucchini bread that can be a dessert or as a sweet part of the main meal.

Makes 2 loaves.

Ingredients:

*2 cups of rice flour
*2 cups of flax meal (golden)
*2 cups of zucchini (shredded)
*1 cup of raisins
*1 cup of apple juice (thawed out from frozen concentrate, not diluted)
*1 cup of hot water
*1/2 cup of yogurt
*1 tablespoon of vanilla extract
*2 teaspoons of baking soda
*1 teaspoon of salt
*1 teaspoon of cinnamon (ground)

Directions:

Prep: Preheat oven to 350 degrees Fahrenheit. Spray 2 loaf pans with cooking spray.

In a bowl, combine the 2 cups of rice flour, 2 cups of golden flax meal, 2 teaspoons of baking soda, 1 teaspoon of salt with the teaspoon of ground cinnamon. In a separate bowl, combine the cup thawed apple juice concentrate with the cup of hot water, 1/2 cup of yogurt, and the tablespoon of vanilla extract. Stir in the 2 cups of shredded zucchini and the cup of raisins. Gradually add the dry ingredients and mix well. Divide between the 2 loaf pans and back for a little over an hour. Cool completely in pan before removing.

Bagels

These bagels are good by themselves or as a sandwich for breakfast, lunch or supper or as a bread with a full meal.

Makes a dozen bagels.

Ingredients:

*2 cups of spelt flour (whole)
*2 cups of spelt flour (white)
*1 cup of milk
*1 packet of yeast
*2 eggs - divided
*1 tablespoon of salt + 1 teaspoon
*1 tablespoon of olive oil
*1 teaspoon of sugar

Directions:

Pour the milk into a saucepan and heat to luke warm. Stir in the packet of yeast. In a bowl, add the yeast milk along with 1 egg, and 1 tablespoon of olive oil and mix. In a separate bowl, mix the 2 cups of whole spelt flour with the 2 cups of white spelt flour and the teaspoon of salt and teaspoon of sugar. Mix in with the wet ingredients to form the dough. Cover the bowl with a cloth and allow rising for about 45 minutes. Preheat the oven to 400 degrees Fahrenheit. Sprinkle a flat surface with flour and coat your hands with flour, pour the dough onto the floured surface and "knead" the dough. Pull apart into a dozen lumps. Roll each dough lump into a rope and form a "ring" the size of a bagel. Add water to a large pot and add the tablespoon of salt. Bring the water to a boil and drop in the bagels, doing one at a time. Boil for 2 minutes. Beat the remaining egg. Remove the bagel and put on a baking sheet. Do this for every bagel. Brush each bagel with the beaten egg. Bake in the preheated oven until golden brown, about 17 minutes.

Main Dish Recipes for Blood Type AB

Chicken Curry

This dish is a one dish meal, or have other side dishes with it.

Makes 4 servings.

Ingredients:

*5 cups of potatoes (quartered)
*3 cups of tomatoes (canned, chopped)
*2 chicken breasts (skinned, boneless and chunked)
*2 cups of onions (chopped)
*1/2 teaspoon of garlic (minced)
*1 bay leaf
*1 vegetable bullion
*1/8 teaspoon of cumin (ground)
*1/8 teaspoon of ginger (ground)
*1/8 teaspoon of paprika
*1/8 teaspoon of cayenne chili pepper
*1/8 teaspoon of turmeric
*olive oil
*salt and pepper

Directions:

Add a little olive oil to a skillet and turn to medium heat. Add the 2 chunked chicken breasts and cook until white. Put the cooked chicken along with the 5 cups of potatoes (quartered), 3 cups of tomatoes (canned, chopped), 2 cups of onions (chopped), 1/2 teaspoon of garlic (minced), 1 vegetable bullion, 1/8 teaspoon of cumin (ground), 1/8 teaspoon of ginger (ground), 1/8 teaspoon of paprika, 1/8 teaspoon of cayenne chili pepper, 1/8 teaspoon of turmeric and the dashes of salt and pepper and stir. Add the bay leaf. Pour enough hot water to cover the food with about an inch over the top. Turn heat to high and stir while it cooks for 15 minutes. Turn heat to low and simmer, covered, for another 15 minutes. Stir often. Dish is done when the potatoes are soft and tender.

Turkey Burgers

These great burgers work well as a sandwich or as a meat with the main meal.

Makes 4 servings.

Ingredients:

*1 pound of turkey (ground)
*1/2 cup of water
*1 teaspoon of lemon zest
*1 teaspoon of chicken broth
*1 teaspoon of lemon juice
*1/2 teaspoon of sage
*1/2 teaspoon of salt
*1/2 teaspoon of ginger (ground)
*couple dashes of hot sauce

Directions:

Add the turkey in a bowl and combine with the 1/2 cup of water, teaspoon of lemon zest, teaspoon of chicken broth, teaspoon of lemon juice and the dashes of hot sauce. In a cup add the 1/2 teaspoons of ground ginger, sage and salt and mix, then sprinkle into the turkey, and with hands mix well. Form into 4 quarter pound patties and cook until well done in a frying pan, grill or under the broiler, about 7 minutes on each side.

Savory Chicken and Wild Rice

This main dish recipe features the wholesome goodness of wild rice with savory herbs and mushrooms to make it as filling, as it is delicious.

Makes 4 servings.

Ingredients:

* 1 1/2 pounds of ground chicken
*4 cups of maitake mushrooms (sliced)
*2 1/2 cups of water
*1 cup of wild rice
*1 1/2cup of chicken broth
*1/2 cup of onion (chopped)
*1/2 cup of celery (chopped)
*2 tablespoons of cornstarch
*2 tablespoons of soy sauce
*1 tablespoon of parsley flakes
*1 tablespoon of basil (dried)
*1 teaspoon of oregano (ground)
*1/2 teaspoon of sage (ground)
*1/2 teaspoon of marjoram
*1/2 teaspoon of rosemary

Directions:

Pour 2 cups of water into a saucepan, add the wild rice, and bring to a boil on high heat. Cover the pan, turn to low, and simmer for 45 minutes. After the rice is cooked place a non-stick skillet on medium high heat and add the remaining 1/2 cup of water. Stir in the 4 cups of sliced maitake mushrooms, 1/2 cup of chopped onion, and the 1/2 cup of chopped celery. Cook and stir for 5 minutes. Pour the 1 1/2 cup of chicken broth into a bowl and mix in the 2 tablespoons of corn starch, 2 tablespoons of soy sauce, tablespoons of parsley flakes, dried basil, teaspoon of ground oregano, 1/2 teaspoons of ground sage, marjoram, and rosemary. Pour into the cooked mushrooms and bring mixture to a boil on medium high. Add the 1 1/2 pounds of ground chicken and the rice. Stir and cook, it will thicken as it cooks. This dish is cooked when the chicken is no longer pink.

Side Dish Recipes for Blood Type AB

Basmati Rice

Sometimes a meal needs a good side dish of flavorful rice and this recipe fits the bill.

Makes 4 servings.

Ingredients:

*2 cups of chicken broth
*1 1/2 cup of basmati rice (uncooked)
*1/2 cup of water
*1/4 cup of onion
*4 tablespoons of butter
*1 teaspoon of salt
*1/2 teaspoon of turmeric
*1/2 teaspoon of garlic (minced)
*1/2 teaspoon of lemon juice.

Directions:

Add the 4 tablespoons of butter to a saucepan and heat on medium to melt the butter. Add the 1/4 cup of onions and sauté. Stir in the 1/2 teaspoon of minced garlic. Add the rice and stir for another 2 minutes. Pour in the 1/2 cup of water, teaspoon of salt, and the 1/2 teaspoon of turmeric and turn the heat to high. Stir constantly until the mixture comes to a boil, and then reduce heat to low and simmer, covered for another 20 minutes. Turn heat off and let it sit for 5 minutes. Place in a serving dish and sprinkle with the 1/2 teaspoon of lemon juice, fluff to mix and serve.

Risotto Tomato Rice

This is a delicious Italian side dish rich in basil and it is absolutely tasty.

Makes 4 small servings or 2 large.

Ingredients:

*4 Roma tomatoes (peeled, seeded and diced)
*3 3/4 cups of tomato juice
*1 cup of Arborio rice
*1/2 cup of mozzarella cheese (grated)
*1/2 cup of basil (fresh chopped)
*1/4 cup of onion (chopped)
*1/4 cup of white wine
*3 tablespoons of butter
*2 teaspoons of garlic (minced)
*2 teaspoons of olive oil
*1/2 teaspoon of salt

Directions:

Add the 2 teaspoons of olive oil to a saucepan and turn to medium heat. Stir in the 1/4 cup of onions and sauté. Add the 2 teaspoons of minced garlic, stir, and cook for another minute. Stir in the cup of Arborio rice and stir for 2 minutes. Pour in the 1/4 cup of white wine and 3/4 cup of the tomato juice. Cook and stir until the rice absorbs all the liquid. Turn the heat to low and add the remainder of the 3 cups of tomato juice and stirring occasionally; cook until the rice is tender enough to eat. Turn the heat to meduim, add the diced roma tomatoes, 1/3 cup of shredded mozzarela cheese, and stir until the cheese melts completely. Turn the heat off and stir in the 1/2 cup of fresh chopped basil and the 1/2 teaspoon of salt. Serve while hot.

Conclusion

Please feel free to modify the recipes within this book, as cooking is like art, it changes with the user. Each recipe, though slated for one particular blood type, may be crossed over as good fits for the other blood types. The best thing to do is to memorize the allowable foods and avoidable foods for your particular blood type and make your own judgments on the recipes. Always seek the advice of your own health care provider before starting any new diet routine. Make sure you are getting all the nutrients your body needs in your diet.

Milton Keynes UK
Ingram Content Group UK Ltd.
UKHW020654221024
2310UKWH00044B/375

9 781631 877902